I want to go to Lithuania
or

How to have Fun with your Aging Parents

I want to go to Lithuania
or
How to have Fun with your Aging Parents

Christina Britton Conroy
M.A., C.M.T., L.C.A.T.

Black Lyon Publishing, LLC

I WANT TO GO TO LITHUANIA
OR
HOW TO HAVE FUN WITH YOUR AGING PARENTS

Our books may be ordered through your local bookstore or by
visiting the publisher:

www.BlackLyonPublishing.com

Black Lyon Publishing, LLC
PO Box 567
Baker City, OR 97814

ISBN: 978-1-934912-77-5
Library of Congress Control Number: 2017936840

Published and printed in the United States of America.

Illustrated by Larry Conroy.

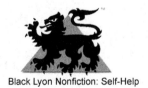

Black Lyon Nonfiction: Self-Help

Dedicated to my husband and perfect life partner, Larry Conroy. When I first conceived this manual, Larry drew two sample cartoons. We never dreamed that he would become ill with Parkinson's and lose his ability to draw. With the help of art therapist Lucia Cristina Hernandez, Larry was able to choose 11 old cartoons from his files, and complete this book.

Special thanks to Betty Anne Crawford at Books Crossing Borders, and my agents Donna Eastman and Gloria Koehler at Parkeast Literary for their faith and candor, sharing their personal caregiving experiences.

TABLE OF CONTENTS

INTRODUCTION

Several years ago, I worked as a recreational therapist in an attractive nursing home. My workweek was Tuesday through Saturday, and I liked Saturdays best. They were quiet.

Every day, two hundred residents on four floors were fed, dressed, and medicated. But on Saturdays there were no podiatrists clipping toenails, psychiatrists adjusting psychotropic medications, medical doctors listening to hearts and lungs, dentists replacing lost dentures, frustrated social workers arguing on telephones, or nursing supervisors instructing new nurses' aides.

There were adult visitors every day, but most Saturdays, the adults were accompanied by children. Quiet or noisy, they burst like merry beams of sunshine through heavy fog, bringing light and health through the sterile hallways.

On Saturdays I was the only recreation staffer on duty and I attempted to entertain all two hundred patients. After lunch a local minister came to the main day room and taught a Bible study class. I took other residents into the dining room to play BINGO.

One Saturday afternoon, a withdrawn little woman got into the elevator with the other residents. She shuffled on terry cloth slippers with jagged holes cut out for her bunions.

Against her worn cotton smock she clutched a teddy bear. Her thin gray hair lay flat against her cheeks, and her pale blue eyes held a vacant stare. She moved to the side of the elevator, and silently waited. Since she was always disoriented and never participated in activities, I was thrilled to see her join the group.

I gently touched her arm. "Mary, it's so good to see you. Do you want to go Bible study or BINGO?" I asked.

Without looking up, she replied, "I want to go to Lithuania."

After stifling a smile and apologizing that we couldn't go to Lithuania that day, I was tempted to take her downstairs with the other residents. Good judgment won out. I led her out of the elevator and helped her shuffle back to her room. Mary did not have enough concentration to enjoy either Bible study or BINGO.

I knew she would sit still for two minutes, fidget, and walk out. Another already overworked staffer would have to leave his/her post, race after her, and take her back upstairs. I felt sorry I was only one person, and had to leave Mary while I collected the 40 other residents who wanted to play BINGO.

I also felt that Mary was all right. She knew what she wanted. She might have known she couldn't really go to Lithuania. From time to time, she may have believed she was in Lithuania. Her mind had taken her away from the unpleasant reality of a nursing home into a pleasant dream-reality.

Another sweet, rosy-cheeked resident sat in her wheelchair next to scrubbed white walls under harsh florescent lights, smiled brightly, and invited me into her garden for tea. She described her flowers and the feel of spring sunshine. It was lovely.

Some clinicians believe that dementia/Alzheimer's patients need constant reality orientation—that they need to be dragged out of their dream worlds, reminded who they are and where they are. Other clinicians practice Naomi Feil's Validation Therapy, trusting that the mind will take a sad person to a place of happiness and peace—a better place than a nursing home.

Medical science has discovered no cures and or even preventatives for dementia/Alzheimer's-related illnesses.

New medications promise to slow the deterioration, but nothing more. Those caring for demented individuals often feel confused, distressed, and desperate. Nothing is more painful than watching the mind of a loved one slowly disappear, leaving only the shell of a body.

A demented person may look perfectly normal, but no longer recognize himself and the world around him. Every caregiver must decide how to care for their deteriorating loved one. I believe that a demented person who imagines himself in beautiful, make-believe surroundings is wise.

I see no benefit in forcing a demented person to give up a pleasant dream reality in favor of an unpleasant real reality. Severely demented individuals, happy in their dream worlds, can sometimes be easier to care for than lucid individuals who are totally aware of and very unhappy with their real life conditions.

Lucid, elderly individuals may feel they have lost their place in the world. With your help, they can discover a new passion, or rekindle an old one, and find real pleasure in their day-to-day lives. This book is about understanding these folks and having fun.

The adventure begins now!

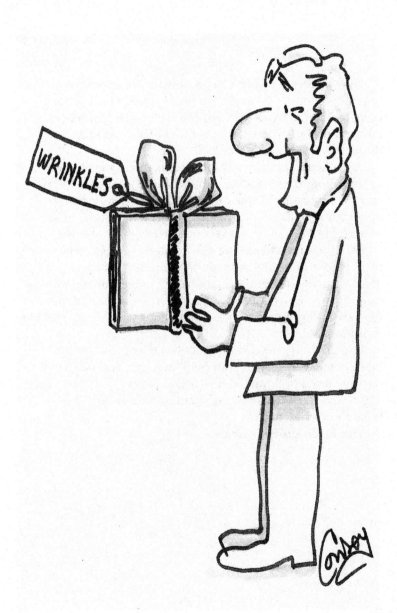

CHAPTER ONE
Old Age: A Gift with a Downside

Much like Pandora's Box, old age is a gift with a downside. Those who are blessed with long life will inevitably see their minds and bodies start to wear out. Life happens. This is part of it. Lucky retirees enjoy good health and have sufficient incomes to cover daily needs. They have friends and family close enough to provide company and emotional support.

Lifelong interests plus new hobbies or second careers can keep these older adults feeling busy and useful until the end of their days. Worldwide tourism booms because of affluent gray-haired travelers wishing to explore the globe. For these folks, old age can truly be what all those TV commercials call, "The Golden Years."

As a Certified Music Therapist, Licensed Creative Arts Therapist, and former Senior Center Director, my work takes me to a variety of medical and social service venues. Among my nursing home patients was an affluent society matron, widowed with adult children, who had enjoyed all the best life had to offer.

Ninety-three and wheelchair-bound, she took an avid interest in everything I offered. She enjoyed watching old and new movies, discussing theatre, literature, and acting in the radio plays I wrote with the patients. Since she had toured the world, she enjoyed travel films, reminiscing about her own experiences, and imaging herself in exotic places.

As we age, we change for better and worse. Gaining

wisdom is wonderful, but losing agility and memory can be devastating. If we can use that wisdom to keep our sense of humor and stay busy, we can adjust and move through the changes very well. Without humor and a strong sense of self, the aging process can be a cruel thief, robbing us of good looks, mobility, sharp eyes, and ears.

Financial concerns can make life hard at any age. If pensions and/or social security are not enough to provide a comfortable lifestyle, if aging siblings and friends have all died, and grown children moved away, the feelings of loss can be devastating.

Medical science is keeping us alive longer, but doing little to make those extended years happy and productive. We all smile at TV news broadcasts covering the latest centenarians. These elderly birthday boys or girls appear to be sweet and kind. Unfortunately, they are often monosyllabic and wheelchair-bound. We cringe watching aging individuals get strapped into wheelchairs, then warehoused along the corridors of nursing homes waiting to die.

Those of us with an aging loved one at home race to bookstores and surf the net hungry for the latest updates on the American healthcare system. Understanding differences between Medicare and Medicaid, how to spend down an aging person's capital, the availability of home health aids, Meals on Wheels, and other services is complex, but vital. Every caregiver must either understand ever-changing government benefits, or work closely with a Certified Social Worker who does. Few books and websites deal with an elderly person's quality of life beyond basic physical needs.

This book does just that. It is a simple, step-by-step manual that can help you and your aging parent, relative, or friend enjoy life by discovering or rediscovering gratifying activities. These activities can be as simple as joining a sing-a-long, or as complex as learning electrical repair.

Every person on the planet enjoys doing something.

For thirty years I have worked with vibrantly healthy elders and the frail elderly. I have counseled and been counseled by hundreds of wise, amusing, elderly men and women, all concerned with some old-age disability.

Whatever their affliction, many have looked stern, pointed a finger, and commanded, "Christina, never grow old!"

My usual response is to smile, give them a hug, and say, "But, I want to grow old. Very old! It sure beats the alternative."

They usually laugh with me. Most elderly people are grateful to be alive. Those few who suffer from clinical depression or chronic pain, truly, and perhaps reasonably, wish for death. These individuals need serious medical and/ or psychiatric attention, right now!

My father died at the age of ninety-two. When people asked me what he died of, I replied, "He died from being ninety-two. He wore out." At the time of his death, my father and I were at peace with each other. The journey to that peace was sometimes heartbreaking. At other times, it was a joy.

You are probably reading this book because you care for an elderly parent, relative, or friend. To simplify my writing, I will refer to these elderly loved ones as your "parent," or "he." If your parent has a safe, comfortable, and fulfilling lifestyle, God bless! May he live long and stay happy. If your parent is no longer capable of caring for himself, feels in some way unfulfilled, unhappy, is self-abusive, a danger to himself or others, this book can help you.

You and your parent may be best friends or virtual strangers with little in common. As a child, you may have been close to your parent. He may have watched over you, encouraged you, and taught you that you were special and loved. If your parent was distant, he may still have loved you, but lacked the nurturing skills to show you that love.

Financial worries, health problems, or circumstances having nothing to do with you, may have determined how your parent related to you, and to the rest of the world. However good or bad your relationship is right now, it can improve, once you have identified these Three Truths:

1. Your Parent's Basic Personality Type
2. Your Relationship to your Parent
3. What your Parent Needs to Feel Validated and Whole

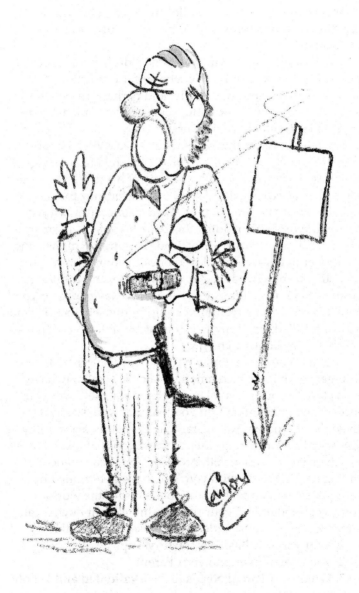

CHAPTER TWO
The Four Dysfunctional Parent Types

In my experience, there are four dysfunctional parent types. Does one of them sound like your parent?

Parent Type 1: Stuck in a rut

"My mother's only seventy-eight. She's healthy, but all she wants to do is get her hair done and play BINGO. She sits around the house all day watching soap operas, and it's driving me crazy. What can I do to make her life more interesting?"

Parent Type 2: Self-isolating

"I'm very worried about Dad. He's eighty-three, and he used to be the life of the party. Now most of his buddies have passed away and he won't even pick up the phone. He's so unhappy. There's a lovely senior citizens' center down the street, but he says he doesn't want to be around, 'Those old people.' He won't go anywhere. What can I do for him?"

Parent Type 3: Dangerously independent

"My mom is eighty-nine, half-blind, deaf, and lame, but still insists on doing everything by herself. She refuses to get rid of her clutter, and I'm afraid she'll burn the house down.

She could fall crossing the street and hurt herself. I'm afraid to leave her alone, but I have to go to work. She won't let anyone else help her. What can I do?"

Parent Type 4: Unreasonably demanding

"I do everything for Dad, but it's never enough. He hates feeling useless, but his arthritis is so bad, he can hardly walk. He's mad at his condition, so he yells at me. I try not to take it personally, but some days, it's hard not to yell back at him. I try to balance my job, my husband, my kids, and my father, but it's too much for one person. If I'm fifteen minutes late, or buy Dad the wrong brand of peanut butter, he starts yelling. He won't allow a home attendant into the house, so what can I do?"

Day after day, frustrated people come to me asking questions, begging for help with their aging parents.

Sometimes the solutions are simple. Often, they are not.

Elderly people with few interests, poor health, and meager finances, who cannot, or choose not to keep busy, can find old age to be confining and miserable.

If they had very few interests when they were young and healthy, and are no longer well enough to do even those few things, they may feel like they have no life at all. The career homemaker who no longer has a spouse or children at home, may feel useless and unwanted. The postman who used to go bowling every Friday night, but can no longer lift heavy mailbags and bowling balls, may feel he has no reason to go on living.

One of my nursing-home patients worked for thirty years as a welder. Every night, for those thirty years, this man came home from the welding shop, got a beer from the refrigerator, and fell asleep in front of the TV. He had no family and no interests outside of his work. Now that he was crippled with arthritis and could no longer move without assistance, he was bitter, angry, and felt he had no life at all.

Eventually, I discovered a passion he did not realize he had. Hour-after-hour, for thirty years, in his welding shop, he had played the radio. He knew hundreds of popular songs, band leaders, and singers. Sitting in a large room with other nursing-home patients, listening to vintage recordings, he was able to lead musical reminiscing sessions.

Sharing his expertise, talking about the music and musicians, he felt smart and important. The other patients enjoyed sharing their memories while listening to the music of their youth.

Exercise: The Four Dysfunctional Parent Types

Which parent type(s) best describes your parent?

_____ **Parent Type 1: Stuck in a rut.** Explain why:

_____ **Parent Type 2: Self-isolating.** Explain why:

_____ **Parent Type 3: Dangerously independent.** Explain why:

_____ **Parent Type 4: Unreasonably demanding.** Explain why:

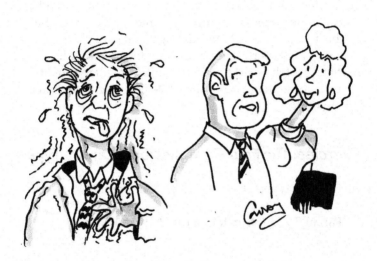

CHAPTER THREE
Defining your Relationship to your Parent

To help your aging parent enjoy the rest of his life, you must understand these five things:

1. How does your parent see himself? Does he think that he is:
- Physically strong, smart, self-sufficient, and able to take care of himself?
- Physically and emotionally weak, overwhelmed by day-to-day chores, needing assistance with every little thing?
- Physically and emotionally healthy, but needing some help, some of the time?

2.   How do you see your parent? Do you think he is:
- Physically strong, smart, self-sufficient, and able to take care of himself?
- Physically and emotionally weak, overwhelmed by day-to-day chores, needing assistance with every little thing?
- Physically and emotionally healthy, but needing some help, some of the time?

3.   How do you see yourself? Do you think you are:
- Physically strong, smart, self-sufficient, with enough spare time to take charge, and do everything for him?
- Physically and emotionally weak, overwhelmed by your own needs, and unable to help him?

• Physically and emotionally strong, with some spare time, so you can help him some of the time?

4. How does your parent see you? Does he think you are:
• Physically strong, smart, self-sufficient, and able to take care of him?
• Physically and emotionally weak, overwhelmed by your own needs, and unable to help him?
• Physically and emotionally strong enough to help him with some things, some of the time?

5. What are the moments in your history that define your relationship to your parent?
• Make a list of your strongest memories of your parent. These can be special occasions, like birthdays or graduations, day-to-day conversations while washing dishes or driving to the supermarket, playing catch in the backyard, or a hundred other memories.

• Without judging these memories, analyze them, attaching an emotion to each one. This will help you understand how you feel about your parent, and your present, immediate gut reactions to his words and actions.

• If you remember a gentle, nurturing parent, he may elicit gentle, nurturing feelings from you.

• If you remember an angry, tyrannical parent, he may elicit angry feelings from you.

Whether your parent is Type 1: Stuck in a rut,   Type 2: Self-isolating, Type 3: Dangerously independent, Type 4: Unreasonably demanding, or a combination of all four, studying the questions above can help you understand your feelings and better relate to him.
If he was over-controlling and abusive when you were young and helpless, you may harbor a deep-seated need for revenge. Now that you are an adult, you may wish to control

and even abuse him.

If he was a sweet and supportive parent, you may wish to be sweet and supportive in return, helping him the way he helped you.

Some adult children feel they need to control their parents, even if their parents are doing just fine the way they are.

In the case of Parent Type 1: Stuck in a rut, the mom who only wants to get her hair done, play BINGO, and watch soap operas, may best be left alone. While adult children must sometimes role-reverse, becoming parents to our parents, we must never forget that our parents are adults.

We must treat them with the same respect we would treat any other adult. If this mom is truly content spending her days doing what she is doing, if she poses no danger to herself or others, and if there is money enough to support her habits, the problem belongs to her adult child and not to her. Sometimes elderly people know exactly what is best for them and just need to be left alone.

Even if this mom was an over-controlling parent, her adult child doesn't need to follow the tradition and become over-controlling, now that the roles are reversed.

Unfortunately, Parent Types 2: Self-isolating, 3: Dangerously independent, or 4: Unreasonably demanding can sometimes endanger themselves and others. They may need different kinds of compassionate control. Their adult children may need to seem cruel, and go against their parents' wishes in order to keep them safe from harm.

Exercise: Defining your Relationship to your Parent

Does your parent think he is:

____ Physically strong, smart, self-sufficient, and able to take care of himself?

____ Physically and emotionally weak, overwhelmed by day-to-day chores, needing assistance with every little thing?

____ Physically and emotionally healthy, but needing some help, some of the time?

Explain why:

Do you think your parent is:

____ Physically strong, smart, self-sufficient, and able to take care of himself?

____ Physically and emotionally weak, overwhelmed by day-to-day chores, needing assistance with every little thing?

____ Physically and emotionally strong enough to do some things for himself some of the time?

Explain why:

Do you think you are:

____ Physically strong, smart, self-sufficient, with enough spare time to take charge and do everything for him?

____ Physically and emotionally weak, overwhelmed by your own needs and unable to help him?

____ Physically and emotionally strong, with some spare time so you can help him some of the time?

Explain why:

Does your parent think you are:

_____ Physically strong, smart, self-sufficient and able to take care of him?

_____ Physically and emotionally weak, overwhelmed by your own needs and unable to help him?

_____ Physically and emotionally strong enough to help him with some things some of the time?

Explain why:

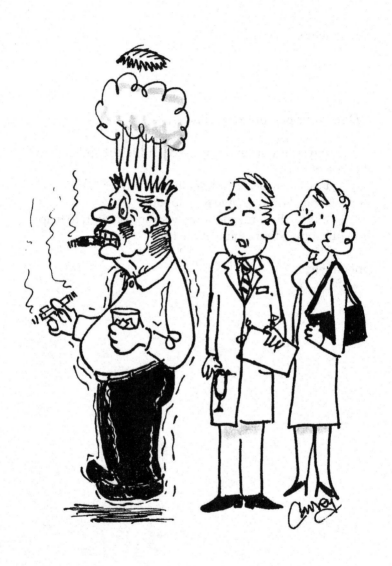

CHAPTER FOUR
Deciding what your Parent Needs

If your parent is Type 2, 3, or 4, please ask yourself:

6. What does my parent want for himself?
7. What does my parent think he needs?
8. Are those wants and needs realistic and possible?
9. What do I think my parent needs?
10. What is/are my parent's passion(s)?
11. What is my relationship to my parent?

Unless you truly understand your relationship to your parent, you can never understand his needs and what is best for him. As a child, you had huge, valid, emotional and physical needs.

If your parent did not fulfill those needs, if he was over-demanding or under-supportive, you may be forty-years-old and still looking for his approval and support. If he was overprotective, you may want him to stop trying to control you. If he was negligent, you may still be waiting for him to become a nurturer.

Even if you are right, and your parent's behavior should change, forget it. He is not perfect and he won't change! You, however, may be wiser and more mature than he is. You can change your expectations of him, relax, see the humor in his imperfections, and allow him to be the normally defective human being he has always been.

Young children often complain about their parents.

Expressing opinions and learning to think for oneself is a normal, healthy part of growing up. Children's complaints can be immature and unfounded, or totally appropriate.

Billy's dad is nicer than my dad because:

• "He lets Billy eat as much candy as he wants."
This complaint is immature. Candy is unhealthy.

• "He cooks Billy dinner. My dad sits watching TV. I have to make my own dinner."
This complaint is appropriate. A young child should not be responsible for shopping, preparing, and/or cooking meals.

• "He helps Billy with his homework. My dad doesn't care if I do my homework."
This is appropriate. A parent should care about his child's schoolwork.

• "He doesn't make Billy do his homework. My dad always checks my homework."
This is immature. To get an education, a child must do his homework.

• "He lets Billy play in the snow without a coat. My dad makes me wear a coat and hat."
This is immature. It is a parent's job to make sure his child is dressed for the weather.

Each of us has a list of things our parent forced us to do, and/or neglected to do for us. These parental behaviors may range from unintentional carelessness to intentional child-abuse, and we may hate him for doing, or neglecting to do those things.

However well or badly your parent treated you, and however valid your complaints against him, now is the time to set those feelings aside, grow up, and become a parent to your parent. Let him stay an immature child set in his ways. He cannot change, but you can. Letting go of your immature anger can allow joy and freedom into your adult life.

I witnessed a dreadful example of adult-child/parent abuse at a nursing home. As the Music Therapist on the psychiatric unit, I was told to expect a new, difficult patient. This was nothing unusual.

Indeed, Ben arrived disoriented, angry, and constantly trying to run away. He didn't know where he was, and could say only a couple of intelligible sentences in a row. He was easily distracted by music, so I was able to calm and entertain him for short periods.

Eventually, we learned Ben had been living in another state with a woman out of wedlock. His adult children disapproved. They told him he was coming home for a short visit.

Instead of visiting his family, then going home to his ladylove, they imprisoned him with us. His family had committed him without his consent.

No wonder he was angry.

After depositing him, his children never came to visit, so I never learned any more family history.

Periodically, his children were contacted and asked to make decisions about his treatment. Every time they said they did not want to be bothered and we should do whatever we thought best.

Some of my colleagues thought his children were callous demons. I tended to agree, but tried to stay nonjudgmental. Knowing nothing about his family history, and knowing that his intelligent adult children hated him, it was possible that he had been an abusive father.

His children may have considered their actions to be righteous retribution. Thinking positively, I credited them for securing a safe, expensive, sanitary environment where their father was well cared for.

We must never judge or second-guess a family history

we don't know, but I hope I never again have to deal with a family that unhappy. I always felt sorry for those adult children. If they never sought counseling or tried to make peace while their father was still alive, their unresolved anger and guilt may have haunted them for the rest of their lives.

Exercise: Deciding what your Parent Needs

What does my parent want for himself?

What does my parent think he needs?

Are those wants and needs realistic and compatible?

What do I think my parent needs?

What is my parent's passion(s)?

What is my relationship to my parent?

What are your strongest memories of your parent?

What emotions do you attach to each memory?

•

I was twenty-seven when my sixty-year-old mother
died of cancer. My brother and I were left to care for our
temperamental, over-controlling, eighty-year-old father.
While grieving for my mother, I was also angry with her for
dying young.

She and I had never been close.

I was left with unresolved mother/daughter issues, and
worst of all, she had deserted us, leaving us to take care of
Dad. She had married a man old enough to be her father. She
knew he would get old and frail.

Taking care of him was supposed to have been her job, not
mine.

Dad was a recently retired psychologist—a brilliant
clinician, loved and respected by his patients and colleagues.

He was financially solvent, physically healthy, and
mentally alert. He was also emotionally needy. He had no
close friends and even discouraged old friends from visiting.

He was a definite Parent Type 2: Self-isolating, and a

partial Parent Type 4: Unreasonably demanding.

I was a singer/actress living from job-to-job, and spending most of my life on the road touring with shows. For the next few years, I carried on with my career, checking in with Dad from motel phones, and seeing him whenever I was home in New York. A couple of years later, my brother married and moved out west. I was left to take care of Dad—alone.

Now, close to ninety, Dad had a comfortable routine, walking around his neighborhood. His bank, grocery store, drugstore, dry cleaners, medical doctor, eye doctor, dentist, and post office were all within a few blocks of his apartment.

There were only two problems:

1. He refused to have his privacy invaded by the presence of a house cleaner. His eyesight wasn't good. The apartment was filthy. His clothes were stained. The kitchen was a disaster.

His favorite food was baked chicken, and I seldom remember seeing his stove and counter tops void of greasy fat. I did some cleaning myself, and eventually persuaded him to let a cleaner in once a month. This wasn't sufficient, but it helped.

2. He was bored, lonely, and wanted me to come over daily. I was struggling to build a career, find a husband, and a start a family of my own. An aging father did not fit into that equation.

My dad had one easy passion. He was from a family of classical musicians, so I marked his *TV Guide*, and encouraged him to watch cultural programs on PBS. Occasionally, we went to concerts together, but like most elderly people, he was fearful of going out at night.

During the day, I was busy taking classes, auditioning, and paying my rent by modeling in fashion shows. Whenever I visited Dad, we shared a cordial dinner. I cleaned his kitchen, then we sat and stared at each other.

We quickly ran out of conversation.

Watching TV together was boring. We had never had fun together when I was growing up, and had no history of activities to fall back on. I didn't know what to do with him.

Although I had not yet written out questions 1 through 11, I instinctively asked myself:

1. How does my parent see himself?
Physically strong, smart, self-sufficient, and able to take care of himself.

2. How do I see my parent?
Physically and emotionally strong enough to do some things for himself.

3. How do I see myself?
Physically and emotionally strong, with enough spare time to help him, some of the time.

4. How does my parent see me?
Physically strong, smart, self-sufficient, and able to take care of him.

5. What moments in your history define your relationship to your parent?
• Age 5: Riding in the front of a grocery store cart he was pushing. Happy memory.
• Constant: Both my parents yelling at each other. Frightening memories.
• Age 12: Running away whenever I saw him coming. Knowing that he'd yell at me, no matter what I was doing. Frightening memory.
• Age 18: Playing poker as a family: Happy memory.
• Age 21: His applauding at my senior voice recital. Bittersweet memory.

6. What does my parent want for himself?
• Total independence to do whatever he wants.
• A lot of attention from me.

7. What does my parent think he needs?

- Total independence.
- My company, to keep him from being lonely.

8. Are those wants and needs realistic and possible?
- No: He is not capable of taking care of all his physical needs.
- No: He needs company, but it doesn't have to be me.

9. What do I think my parent needs?
- A home-attendant cleaning his apartment, doing his laundry, and accompanying him outside, in case he falls and hurts himself.
- To socialize, and be with other people.

10. What is my parent's passion(s)?
Classical Music.

11. What is my relationship to my parent?
Strained. We have never been close, never spoke about personal issues, so now it was hard to start.

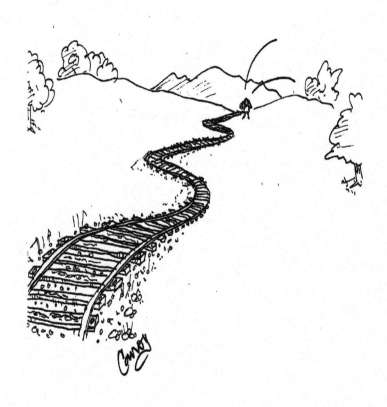

CHAPTER FIVE
Discovering what your Parent Enjoys

My theatrical training had taught me to improvise and use my imagination. These tools served me well.

After weeks of failing to entertain my father, I finally realized there was only one thing he never tired of—talking about himself. His family immigrated to the U.S. in 1905. He studied psychology with the great Carl Jung, had been a studio physician in Hollywood during the 1930s, and an over-aged pilot during WWII.

I had heard these same stories for years, but telling them over and over entertained him, so I devised a plan. I didn't know it, but this basic reminiscing was the start of my work as a Creative Arts Therapist.

Years later, during graduate school training, I was taught that old people with no future gain feelings of self-worth from remembering past accomplishments. Reminiscing is a clinical technique practiced in every competent geriatric facility.

I bought Dad a small cassette tape recorder and a dozen blank tapes. Being a starving actress with little cash on hand, I was constantly in need of homemade gifts and cards for my friends. After dinner, I set up my watercolors, put the tape recorder in front him, and asked him questions. He talked and I painted.

He was easily engaged, and it was simple to lead him from topic to topic. After a couple of hours, I finished a card or caricature. He held a finished tape in his hand and felt happily fulfilled. I still have dozens of hours of his taped stories. Although they may never be played, their creation gave him pleasure. That was an end in itself.

• My dad's passion was talking about himself.
• His passion did not interest me, but I was willing to be bored, in order to please him.
• I painted while he told his stories, and we both stayed entertained.

There are a hundred ways you can entertain your parent and yourself.

Here are a few examples:

Working together you can:

1. Prepare a meal.
2. Go out for a meal.
3. Shop (in stores, from catalogues, or online) for yourselves or others.
4. Sew, knit, paint, sculpt, or otherwise make gifts for family members and friends.
5. Correspond with family members and friends.
6. Write to your congressman.
7. E-mail the President.
8. Google your favorite actor/singer, follow them on Facebook.
9. Build your own Facebook page and find old friends.
10. Make a scrapbook of anything that interests you.
11. Practice or learn a foreign language.
12. Sing or compose songs.
13. Play or listen to music—you can find every variety of music on YouTube.
14. Write a family history or draw a family tree.
15. Play cards, board games, video games, horseshoes, catch, or other simple games—beanbags are sometimes better than balls, because they don't roll.
16. Watch TV or videos.
17. Go to movies, plays, or concerts.

18. Read aloud to each other.

19. Read plays and take all the parts.

20. Put together model airplanes or puzzles.

21. Study travel brochures, Google foreign countries, and plan trips you may never take.

22. Clean out a closet, and decide which items to keep and which to give away.

23. Go through the internet investigating worthy charities that collect used clothing.

Working apart, in the same room, you can do work you need to do: check your e-mail, mend, draw, pay bills, paint your nails, or any of a dozen other things.

While you do those, your parent could:

1. Put a puzzle together.

2. Write a poem to go inside a greeting card you paint.

3. Paint his own greeting card.

4. Design rooms/shelves/wallpaper—you may not need these, but the mental exercise could be terrific.

5. Write out favorite family recipes and dinner menus for his own meals, and/or to give as gifts.

6. Google new recipes.

7. Reminisce, telling stories into a tape recorder.

8. Read aloud.

9. Watch TV, videos or YouTube.

10. Play music, sing songs.

11. Reminisce while listening to vintage records, letting the music trigger memories.

Before you leave for the day, assign him something to think about, or work on, until your next visit. If he doesn't have a reason for living, you may need to invent one for him.

His homework could be:

1. Clean out a drawer or closet.

2. Google long-lost family members.

3. Choose a special memory to go with every vintage song on a re-engineered CD.

4. Write out as many words as he can remember in a foreign language.

5. Plan a week's meals and a shopping list to go with them.

These activities may be too difficult for parents who suffer from dementia or Alzheimer's disease. Most of my patients, who can no longer make conversation still enjoy finishing nursery rhymes and singing songs from their youth.

I say: "Humpty-Dumpty sat on a ..."
And wait for them to say: "... wall."

I say: "Humpty-Dumpty had a great..."
And wait for them to say: "... fall."

I sing: "My bonny lies over the ..."
And wait for them to sing: "... ocean."

I sing: "My bonny lies over the ..."
And wait for them to sing: "... sea."

Hearing old songs like *I've Been Working on the Railroad* and *You are my Sunshine*, Christmas carols and other religious songs can energize sleepy, demented people, start them moving to the music, singing, and playing along on drums and tambourines. Even hostile elders can become happily involved in a song, make eye contact, hold a hand, and enjoy swaying to the beat.

Whenever I meet a caregiver, my first question is always, "What's your parent's favorite song?" The fastest way for me to develop a friendly relationship with a patient is to sing his favorite song.

Since my father's first language was Hungarian, and I never learned that language, I was unable to access his long-term memory with Hungarian nursery rhymes and children's songs.

Exercise: Discovering what your Parent Enjoys

List activities you and your parent could enjoy doing together.

List separate activities you and your parent could do at the same time in the same room.

1. While I do:

   My parent does:

2. While I do:

   My parent does:

3. While I do:

   My parent does:

4. While I do:

   My parent does:

List assignments for your parent to think about, or work on, until your next visit.

•

Visits with my dad stayed busy and amicable. We repeated the same two activities over and over: Listening to classical music and recording his life story.

When his short-term memory started going, serious problems followed. I would call and tell him what time I was arriving. He would forget, and wait by the apartment door buzzer for hours.

When I arrived on time, he was angry, believing I was late. More dangerous was his forgetting to turn off the flame under the teakettle and burning out the bottom.

Every few weeks, I walked in the door with a parcel and Dad asked, "Is that the new teakettle?" It became a bad joke.

Most frightening was the day I visited and found he had melted the back of his polyester jacket by standing too near the flame. It was very obvious he needed supervision.

Since he barely allowed a cleaner inside the apartment, he flatly refused to hire a home attendant.

At this point, I had to rethink my father's Three Truths:

1. Your parent's basic personality type:
He used to be Parent Type 2; Self-isolating, and Parent Type 4: Unreasonably demanding.

Now he had become-Parent Type 3: Dangerously independent.

2. Your relationship to your parent:
Now it was even more strained, and also confused. I had no idea what to do for him or with him.

3. What your parent needs to feel validated and whole:
He needed to feel he was still in control of his life. Memory loss was robbing him of that control.

Our worst day came just as I was lucky enough to get two jobs at once. During the day, I was modeling wedding dresses in a designer's showroom.

Immediately after my last fashion show, I jumped on a train to New Jersey where I was doing a play at night. I got back home near dawn, and tried to sleep quickly in order to get up for my early morning fashion show the next day.

In the middle of this wonderful but hectic routine, I got a call from a police officer. Dad had fallen, broken his hip and was in the emergency room.

They operated that day. The hip surgery was a success, but the anesthetic made him violently ill. He was already very thin. Two days later, he was still unable to eat, constantly writhing, hallucinating, and starving to death.

The overworked nursing staff told me he was, "too sick," for them to deal with.

He needed around-the-clock private nursing, but private nurses needed to be paid daily, in cash, a lot more than I made from my two jobs. Dad had sufficient money in the bank, but I couldn't get at it.

A very kind hospital notary came to Dad's bedside, and had enough of a conversation with him so he could sign over his Power of Attorney. I'm not sure Dad really knew or remembered I was controlling his money and paying his private nurses.

He had always hated spending money on anything, so if he had known, he might have refused their services.

This was the first of several compassionate lies I had to tell my father to insure his safety.

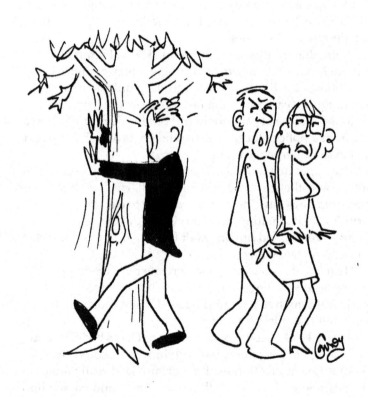

CHAPTER SIX
Compassionate Lies

I hated lying to my father, but had no alternative. I soon learned compassionate lies are necessary. This lie injured no one and possibly saved my father's life.

As soon as he was released from the hospital, his mind cleared enough that he demanded his independence. He was terribly frail, needed round-the-clock home attendants, but refused to hire them. My two jobs were both close to ending, and for about a minute, I considered giving them up and moving in with him. Knowing full well the close confinement would make us hate each other, and knowing he could easily afford to hire professional help, I told him another lie.

Dad remembered paying all kinds of insurance premiums. None of those policies—household-insurance, car-insurance, life-insurance, or malpractice-insurance—covered home nursing.

I lied. I told him they did. He believed me. I warned the home attendants only to accept payment from me, and never from him. I told them to repeat the story that they were being paid by his insurance and warned them, "If you let him pay you, he will fire you."

Again, I hated lying to my father, but I had no alternative. Compassionate lies are necessary. This lie injured no one. It insured my father's safety, and saved my sanity.

My father lived another, mostly pleasant, three years.

Dementia and physical frailties increased until his quiet death at the age of ninety-two. During those last years, he seldom left his apartment. His wonderfully sensitive home attendants understood his need for privacy. They did their work, then kept their ears open while hiding away in a back room letting him think he was alone.

As his memory failed, entertaining him became simpler, but more tedious. He often forgot who I was. At first this made me feel hurt and angry. Soon, I stopped taking it personally, understood that it was his illness, and that it had nothing to do with me.

Some days he was totally lucid and realized whole days had gone by that he couldn't remember. We never spoke about it, but I'm sure his condition made him angry and afraid.

On bad days, he looked at me vacantly. I smiled, reminded him who I was, showed him family photos, and played classical music for him.

Week after week, he enjoyed my visits, and told me how happy I made him. That made me happy. I felt like I was doing him some good. When he died, I felt we were at peace with one another.

•

I continued on with my performing career, thinking I would do the same work forever. Everything changed the Christmas I was hired to sing carols at a nursing home. I took my small Irish harp and entertained a half-dozen residents at a time in several locations around the building.

Unlike singing on a large stage with a faceless audience sitting in the dark, these few, frail people stared vacantly. I started singing *Hark the Herald Angels Sing*, and suddenly, like wilted flowers, they seemed to bloom with new life. Their sagging bodies physically changed. Shouting out the lyrics of the old holiday song, they sat up singing with pure joy. For the first time, I truly realized that music could be much more than just entertainment.

That night changed my life. I applied, auditioned, and was accepted into New York University's Music Therapy Masters Degree program.

At the same time, I started working full-time in a nursing home. I stayed at the home for two years, working with frail-elderly residents, then moved on to a job with well-elderly at a walk-in senior citizens' center. Now, many years later, I am able to help older adults and their younger adult caregivers live fuller lives.

I know how hard it can be for everyone, and how brave everyone needs to be. I also know that a lot of the pain can be transformed into fun.

Even if you have never had fun with your parent, it's not too late to start. You just need some simple tools and imagination.

Exercise

What compassionate lies might you have to tell your parent to keep him safe?

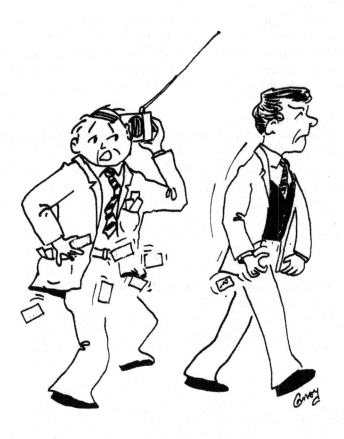

CHAPTER SEVEN
Drum Talk, a Communication Game

Please ask yourself, throughout his life:

1. Was my parent outspoken and dominant, flexible, or submissive and eager to please?

2. Did he enjoy doing for himself, or did he like to be waited on?

3. Did he demand attention, or defer to others?

4. Was he a quick decision-maker, slow and cautious, or afraid of making decisions?

5. Do I enjoy doing for myself, or do I like to be waited on?

6. Do I demand attention, or defer to others?

7. Am I a quick decision-maker, slow and cautious, or afraid of making decisions?

People are complex. You and your parent may be all these things at some time. Thinking about your parent and yourself in those terms can help you to understand what you both want and need, right now.

Even if you think you know the answers to those questions, I suggest you play a game I call Drum Talk. If you happen to have two hand-drums in the house, great. If you don't, two empty cardboard boxes will do nicely.

1. Tell your parent you are going to play a game, and it is going to be fun and easy.

2. Give your parent his drum (or box), then take your own drum and sit across from him.

3. Ask your parent to listen while you play a rhythm, because he is going to play it back to you.

4. When you are sure he is comfortable and listening, play a short, simple rhythm of two or three beats.

5. Carefully study your parent as he listens and plays your rhythm back to you.

6. Repeat the exercise a few times, changing your rhythms, making them easier or harder, to keep his attention, without frustrating him.

7. Then switch—ask your parent to play a rhythm, which you will play back to him.

8. Repeat the game, going back-and-forth until you are able to answer the following questions.

Please ask yourself:
___ Did I play slowly and clearly enough so my parent could hear my rhythms?
___ Were my rhythms too fast and disorganized?
___ Did he easily repeat my rhythms?
___ Was my parent confused by the sounds?
___ Did my parent play back quickly?
___ Did he hesitate before playing back?
___ Did I wait to play my subsequent rhythms until my parent was ready to hear them?
___ Did I rush ahead and catch him by surprise?
___ Did I hesitate before playing, and wait longer than necessary?
___ Did my parent wait patiently until I played my next rhythm?
___ Did he get impatient waiting for me to play?

Now ask yourself:
___ Did my parent play slowly and clearly enough so I could hear his rhythms?
___ Were his rhythms too fast and disorganized?
___ Was I confused by the sounds?

___ Was I able to repeat his rhythms?
___ Did I play back quickly?
___ Did I hesitate before playing back?
___ Did he wait to play his subsequent rhythms until I was ready to hear them?
___ Did he rush ahead and catch me by surprise?
___ Did he hesitate before playing, and wait longer than necessary?
___ Did I wait patiently until he played his next rhythm?
___ Did I get impatient waiting for him to play?

This simple, nonverbal game can quickly define a relationship. If one person thinks and acts much faster than the other, there may be conflict. If the fast person asks a question and the slow person takes too long to think about his answer, the fast person may become impatient and angry. If the slow person cannot quickly understand and respond to the fast person, he may feel embarrassed and inferior.

Tennis players can only volley if they both hit the ball back- and-forth at the same speed. One player will purposely break the volley by hitting faster, or in a new direction. Your parent may not be able to change the speed he speaks and reacts, but you probably can. Carefully listening and watching, you can mirror the speed your parent speaks and acts.

People who already communicate well, love playing Drum Talk. They instinctively act and react at the same speed with similar intensity, and find the game fun to play. Those who have trouble communicating verbally may have even more trouble communicating nonverbally. Practicing this game can result in better overall communication between you both.

I used this game with an elderly couple who were not getting along. The husband, Peter, was healthy, eighty-one, and the retired manager of a prestigious publishing company. Tall and thin, always dressed in a suit and tie, he was soft-spoken and a perfect gentleman. Peter was the child of Hungarian immigrants and grew up during the great depression.

The day he turned fourteen, his father took him out of school so he could get a work permit. He was offered two jobs, and took the one paying pennies more a week: Mail-clerk at the same publishing house he retired from fifty-one years later.

During his long career, Peter read voraciously. He hobnobbed with literary giants, and his personal library of autographed first editions was astounding. Nevertheless, he always felt inferior to scholars who had read those same books in school and received academic degrees.

When I first met Peter, I was the Supervisor of Educational and Recreational Services at a senior citizens' center.

Peter was care-taking his seventy-six-year-old wife, Emma. She had a history of psychiatric and physical problems. She used a walker at home, a wheelchair outside, was demanding and temperamental. They lived near the center, came for lunch and a respite from living in the close confinement of two rooms in a three-story walkup.

Peter would wheel Emma into the center's dining room, get her lunch tray, cut her meat, and do his best to please her. Every time, something displeased her. She started screaming and heaped verbal abuse on her gentle husband. Although Emma was Peter's spouse, she was the equivalent of Parent Type 4: Unreasonably demanding.

My staffers and I devised a plan. The moment the couple arrived in the center, a colleague wheeled Emma away from Peter, into an activity room where she was entertained with other wheelchair-bound center members. She enjoyed the special attention and Peter was free to spend a couple of hours socializing and participating in my music programs, which he loved.

One day, I got Peter and Emma alone, gave them each a hand drum, and told them that they were going to play a game called Drum Talk. Ten minutes of Drum Talk taught me more about their relationship than I would have learned in hours of verbal therapy.

Peter started. He poised his drum, paused, took time to think, looked to Emma for approval, then slowly raised his hand, and beat three slow, soft beats.

Grinning, Emma quickly pounded back his three beats.

He looked startled, watched her, thought for a few moments, raised his hand, and gently played four slow beats.

She pounded back four furious beats, and sat staring, waiting for more.

After Peter had played a few more slow, cautious rhythms, she became angry that he was taking so long.

He tried to play faster, but became flustered.

Then they switched. Enjoying taking control, Emma slammed furiously into her drum, playing wildly. She finally stopped.

Peter could not possible play her rhythm back, and sat looking to me for help.

Emma scolded him for not playing the game.

I calmed her by commending her athletic playing, then explained that her rhythm was too fast and too long for anyone to remember. I asked that her next rhythm be slow and short.

Pleased by my compliment, she played a short, slow rhythm, and Peter easily played it back.

Her next rhythm was faster, and the third so complicated he couldn't possibly play it back.

She scolded him again.

Peter was slow and thoughtful. He needed to take his time and think things through before acting. Emma was impulsive. She thought and moved quickly. It doesn't take a lot of imagination to picture these two opposite personalities dealing with a domestic situation. The next time I had Peter alone, he explained an average morning.

After getting Emma out of bed, helping her on and off her commode, he helped her to stand balanced on her walker while he gave her a sponge bath. He dressed her, helped her brush her teeth, comb her hair, and slowly walked her to the breakfast table.

She sat, waiting for him to bring her pills and morning coffee.

He moved slowly around the kitchen, sorting through her

medications, opening the bottles, and sometimes dropping pills on the floor.

She got restless and scolded him for being slow.

He finally put her coffee mug and pills on the table, then stood waiting for instructions.

He always forgot something, and she told him to get the sugar, or milk, or whatever he had forgotten.

He walked back to the kitchen, brought her the sugar, but forgot the spoon.

She demanded a spoon, and he shuffled back into the kitchen.

She took her spoon, dipped it into the sugar bowl, brought the full spoon to her cup, but her hand shook, and the sugar spilled across the table.

He took a napkin and started wiping up the spilled sugar, before she had gotten any into her coffee.

She started screaming.

Exercise: Drum Talk, a Communication Game

Before playing the game, please ask yourself, throughout his life:

___ Was my parent outspoken and dominant, or flexible, or submissive and eager to please?

___ Did he enjoy doing for himself, or did he like to be waited on?

___ Did he demand attention, or defer to others?

___ Was he a quick decision-maker, slow and cautious, or afraid of making decisions?

___ Am I outspoken and dominant, flexible, or submissive and eager to please?

___ Do I enjoy doing for myself, or do I like to be waited on?

___ Do I demand attention, or defer to others?

___ Am I a quick decision maker, slow and cautious, or afraid of making any decisions?

After playing the game, please ask yourself:

___ Did I play slowly and clearly enough so my parent could hear my rhythms?

___ Was my playing too fast and disorganized?

___ Was my parent confused by the sounds?

___ Was he able to repeat my rhythms?

___ Did my parent play back quickly?

___ Did he hesitate?

___ Did I wait to play my subsequent rhythms until my parent was ready to hear them?

___ Did I rush ahead and catch him by surprise?

___ Did I hesitate before playing and wait longer than necessary?

___ Did my parent wait patiently until I played my next rhythm?

___ Did he get impatient waiting for me to play?

___ Did my parent play slowly and clearly enough so I could hear his rhythms?

___ Was his playing too fast and disorganized?

___ Was I confused by the sounds?

___ Was I able to repeat his rhythms?

___ Did I playback quickly, or hesitantly?

___ Did he wait to play his subsequent rhythms until I was ready to hear them?

___ Did he rush ahead and catch me by surprise?

___ Did he hesitate before playing, and wait longer than necessary?

___ Did I wait patiently until he played his next rhythm?

___ Did I get impatient waiting for him to play?

•

Peter had no help around the house, and did everything for Emma. He bathed her, dressed her, fed her, helped her on and off the commode, emptied the commode, washed the dishes, took out the laundry, did the shopping, the cooking, and was on call to her 24/7 without a break. She slept in their one bed, while he curled, uncomfortably, into the short sofa. Emma's frail health restricted her actions and kept her from making normal life decisions. She was a quick thinker and mover. Waiting for her slow-moving husband to do her bidding made her feel helpless and angry.

In order to help Emma and Peter, I asked him to tell me Emma's Three Truths, changing the word "parent," to "wife."

1. Your wife's basic personality type
Parent Type 4: Unreasonably demanding

2. Your relationship to your wife
Strained.

3. What your wife needs to feel validated and whole
Constant attention and pleasurable activities that keep her mind occupied.

Next, Peter answered questions 1 through 11, again changing the words, "my parent," to "my wife."

1. How does my wife see herself?
Physically weak, but smart, self-sufficient, and mostly able to take care of herself.

2. How do I see my wife?
Physically and emotionally weak. I have to do everything for her.

3. How do I see myself?
Physically and emotionally strong enough to help her, some of the time.

4. How does my wife see me?
Physically and emotionally weak. Unable to take care of us both.

5. What moments in your history define your relationship to your wife?
- Birth of our daughters: Happy memories.
- Emma's psychotic episodes: Frightening memories.
- Emma telephoning me at work, interrupting important business: Angry memories.
- Emma embarrassing me at the senior center: Angry memories.

6. What does my wife want for herself?
- Total independence to do whatever she wants.
- A lot of attention from me.

7. What does my wife think she needs?
- Total independence.
- The complete attention of everyone around her.

8. Are those wants and needs realistic and possible?
No: She is not capable of taking care of her physical needs.

No: She needs company, but not constant attention.

9. What do I think my wife needs?
A home attendant seeing to her physical needs, cleaning the apartment, and giving me a break so I can have some peaceful time alone.

10. What are my wife's passion(s)?
TV, crafts projects, BINGO, card games, visits from family and friends.

11. What is my relationship to my wife?
Strained. We had a hard time getting along when she was agile. Now that she can't move very well, it's even worse.

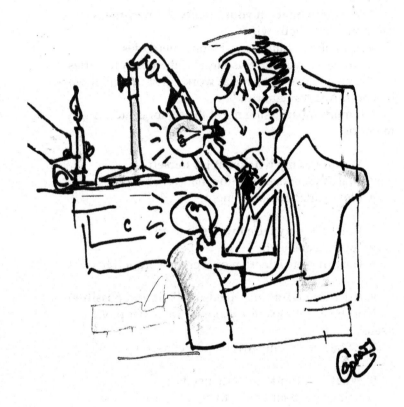

CHAPTER EIGHT
Simple Coping Tools

The first thing I did was to place Peter with a social worker who arranged for a home-attendant to come to their apartment and help out. At first the attendant came for only a few hours a week. Eventually, attendants came seven-days-a-week.

Peter and I worked out an action plan that minimized the stress for both Emma and him. Instead of sitting her at the table, leaving her with nothing to do, then starting to prepare her meal, now he left her in front of the TV or at her crafts table until he finished all his preparations.

Since he usually forgot something in the kitchen, we made lists of all the items that needed to be on the table. He could check the appropriate list before each meal.

Only after the table was completely set with her food on the plate did he bring her to the table. Her need for instant gratification was fulfilled.

She could plow through an entire meal without making him get up, and he could actually sit down and enjoy his own meal.

- Making lists and sticking to routines can be comforting both to your parent and you.
- If your parent has his pills set out in individual containers for each day, he will have an easier time taking the correct medications.

• If he knows he will be taken to the grocery store, launderette, drugstore, etc., on the same day every week, he may not fret about it on other days.

Seventy-three-year-old Maria was overweight, but in good health, and caring for her husband Carlos, who was dying of throat cancer. Carlos was another: Parent Type 4: Unreasonably demanding.

Fourteen years before, Carlos had left Maria for a younger woman. He still lived with the other woman, a nurse who worked an early morning hospital shift. Every day at dawn—rain, sleet, or snow—Maria left the comfort of her apartment and traveled downtown to take care of her husband while his live-in girlfriend was at work.

Maria had been sexually abused as a teenager. She grew up in a household where it was believed that men could do no wrong and women should be treated like servants. She believed that she was totally responsible for her husband's daytime care. Carlos was physically capable of doing a lot of things for himself, but he demanded she wait on him hand and foot. She felt it was her duty to obey him.

The tumor in Carlos's throat allowed him to swallow only thinly pureed liquids. Maria was a good cook and creatively blended tasty fruit drinks, vegetable purees, and cream soups for his lunch.

At breakfast, he insisted on traditional breakfast foods, then scolded that he was bored with the two choices of almost raw egg, or watery hot cereal.

We couldn't think of any alternative breakfast foods, but I suggested that Maria buy a variety of hot cereals, a selection of sweet toppings, and offer him choices.

While choosing between thin wheatina, oatmeal, cream of wheat, cream of rice, with honey, maple syrup, blueberry syrup, raspberry syrup, etc., may not seem exciting to most of us, it worked for Carlos, and relieved Maria's breakfast dilemma.

Carlos's frail health restricted his actions and kept him from making normal life decisions. He felt helpless and angry. Creating choices he could make, like which breakfast cereal to eat, what TV program to watch, or what color shirt to wear, gave him back some lost dignity.

When Carlos was too ill to remain at home, and admitted to the hospital, the doctor was introduced to his wife and girlfriend. The doctor took a moment, said, "Lucky man," and shook hands with both ladies. A few days later, Carlos died with both women at his bedside.

Weary spouses, Maria and Peter, were both in my music therapy group for caregivers.

For the next year, Maria stayed in the group, working through the anger, grief, and love she still felt for her deceased, abusive husband.

Peter became too frail to manage his three-story walkup, but he did not want to leave his old neighborhood. With my urging, he and Emma moved into a specially designed, supportive residence for older adults. There was an elevator and round-the-clock nurses aides taking care of Emma.

Finally, Peter had some time to take care of himself.

Always remember that you are not alone.

Individual counseling and caregiver support groups are everywhere. A phone call to your local hospital, senior center, chamber of commerce, or a glance over the internet can give you all the information you need.

A list of national agencies dedicated to the elderly is in the back of this book.

Exercise: Simple Coping Tools

Which of the following could help you cope with your dysfunctional parent?

____ Engaging a home attendant or other household helper

____ Keeping lists of items that need to be on the dinner table, in the bathroom, etc.

____ Following orderly procedures to see that simple,

everyday tasks have a dependable beginning, middle, and end

___ Scheduling your parent's week in advance so he knows what to expect and not worry he will miss something

___ Offering your parent choices: What to wear, what to eat, which TV program to watch, letting him feel he is in charge

Please write your own:

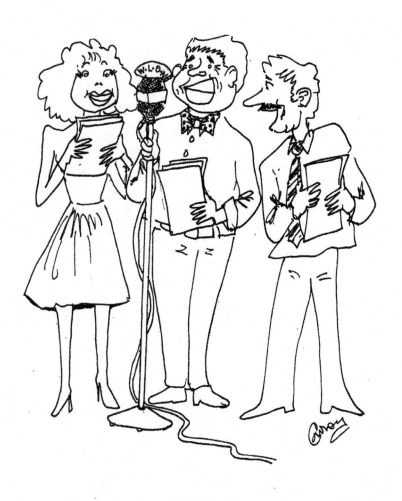

CHAPTER NINE
Discovering your Parent's Passion

- Having a Passion = Life
- Having No Passion = Boredom = Slow Death

Everybody has a passion, but hooking into that passion can be a challenge. It took me months of trying different activities before I realized my father just wanted to talk about himself. If you're lucky, your parent will find his own passion and save you the hassle of finding one for him.

This very thing happened with a tough Irish-American, former saloon owner named Peg. She was a lady in her late seventies living alone in a housing project, lame, widowed, angry, and bored. She came to my senior center to eat lunch, play cards, and complain. Most of the staff dreaded her presence because every word out of her mouth was loud and negative. I assumed the role of Peg's adult child and recorded her Three Truths:

1. Your parent's basic personality type
Parent Type 1: Stuck in a rut.
2. Your relationship to your parent
Strained.
3. What your parent needs to feel validated and whole
I had no idea. I hadn't discovered her passion.

For years, Peg had avoided the seniors' monthly membership meetings, so I was cautiously pleased the first time she stood up to speak. The members had collected a sizable nest-egg and were deciding how to spend it.

Peg wanted the center to buy a pool table. She had been a pool shark in her saloon days, loved playing, but didn't enjoy playing in public pool halls.

The administration did not want a pool table in the building. I had no feelings about it one way or the other, but I was interested, watching Peg passionately describing the virtues of a pool table. For the next few weeks, she went from member to member and staffer to staffer pleading her cause. Eventually, she won the members' votes, was handed their money, and went shopping.

Reporting back on her visits to pool table vendors was very entertaining. She knew the brand of table she wanted, what she thought she should pay for it, and she wouldn't settle for anything else.

The pool table arrived at the senior center to much pomp and circumstance. It became not only Peg's emotional resurrection, but the revival of a dozen dozy senior center men who stood up from their card tables for the first time in years. I was pleased when pool tournaments started self-generating, not only between the seniors, but between the seniors and local high school kids.

Peg and other center members starting teaching lessons. She even researched tournament rules, copied them out in large print, and posted them. She was still tough and loud, but now she joked and laughed a lot more than she complained.

If you don't know your parent's passion, find out what he did for fun when he was young and healthy. If he was athletic but can no longer do his favorite activity full-out, he might enjoy a modified version. A lightweight bowling set, portable basketball hoop, or beanbag toss can keep some elderly jocks happy for hours at a time.

While I was still working at the nursing home, I met Dennis. He was a quiet, wheelchair-bound patient only in his late seventies, but disabled with numerous chronic conditions. For months I had see him sitting in a corner, reading mysteries, not talking, and avoiding my group activities. When I had time to chat with him, he was always pleasant, made small talk, but never let himself get into a real conversation. His Three Truths were:

1. Your parent's basic personality type
Parent Type 2: Self-isolating.
2. Your relationship to your parent
Pleasant but distant.
3. What your parent needs to feel validated and whole
I had no idea. I hadn't discovered his passion.

One day I brought in a miniature electric piano about fourteen inches long. A few of the residents found it amusing, so I showed it to Dennis. He was not musical, but he was fascinated by its mechanics and played with it for a long time. Guessing that he liked gadgets, I next let him play with a handheld cassette tape recorder. He loved it. I had already started recording life histories from some of the residents, and asked Dennis to be my official sound man.

He accompanied me while another charming resident, suffering with Lou Gherig's Disease, recalled his days as a waiter at Harlem's Cotton Club. A woman resident, with little short-term, but great long-term memory, told us about growing up in a poor Irish village. She had to wait three years for her first communion, because there weren't enough white dresses to go around.

Dennis's natural curiosity made him a good interviewer. He liked the stories, but he loved the show biz. Soon, he was keeping the tape recorder by his bed and setting off on his own. There was an easily accessible PA system, and he became a roving reporter, going to all four floors, collecting gossip from the nurses. First thing every morning, we heard the PA click on and, "Good morning! This is Dennis, your ACU weatherman." He gave the weather report, menus, activity list for the day, and any personal interest stories he had collected.

I started a radio play-writing group, and Dennis was

the first to join. Radio format is perfect for elderly actors because they do not have to look the parts or memorize their lines.

They do need clear speaking voices, steady enough fingers to turn pages, and good enough eyesight to read large print. It was amazingly hard to find nursing home residents who had all three abilities.

Dennis contributed this charming recollection from his youth. I recorded it, transcribed it, and used it in one of our plays: *A Place for all Seasons.*

Dennis: *When I was a boy on the farm, we didn't have too much to do. We had no money to go anywhere with, and the pastime was just to hang around in a group. We'd have a few jokes and laughs, and if we had a chance, we got a jug of corn whisky. We passed that around, and we all got feeling good together on a Saturday night. That was what we called a big time.*

Now, when it came to the ladies, we each had our own favorite girlfriend. Some of the girls did, and some didn't. Those that didn't, didn't have too much fun. Those that did were the ones that everyone wanted to go out with. We didn't have many places to go. We maybe had one car amongst the group, and everyone couldn't go in that.

The farmers, in those days, used to cut the tall grass, and make hay out of it. We'd pile up the hay into haystacks. Each one of us would take his girlfriend out into the fields, and dig our way into those haystacks. From there on in, it was everyone for himself. It was a great thing in the good old days. If you don't believe me, go into the country and try it!

Everyone has a story. Often the simplest people, who struggled to survive, have the most interesting stories. Everyone likes talking about themselves, so try recording your parent's life stories, and transcribing them. (If the stories don't happen to be quite true, who cares?)

Using the nursing home residents' own stories, we wrote and performed three radio plays during the two years I worked at the home. Once, we even packed the actors, wheelchairs, microphones, and all onto a bus so they could "go on tour" and perform at another nursing home. Our first play was a mystery: *The Case of the Missing Dentures.*

Next came: *Call us Lucky: Immigration stories based on the real experiences of the elderly actors or their parents.*

Our last play was: *A Place for all Seasons.* This fictional story started in the present, with a little boy (played by a short old lady), finding a fiddle in his grandmother's attic. His grandmother told him their family history, using the fiddle and fiddle music as the centerpiece for important historic and family events. It began with the Armistice of World War I, and ended back in the present, with the little boy wanting to learn to play the fiddle.

Twelve geriatric actors played thirty-six different roles.

My method of writing these plays was rewarding, but labor intensive. The actors made up the story they wanted to tell, broke up the story into short scenes, then picked the character(s) they wanted to play. Scene by scene, sitting in a circle, they improvised dialogue into a tape recorder. I took the recording, transcribed it, and presented them with large-print scripts of their own words.

One of the funniest scenes created this way was about five women coming to the funeral of the man they all thought was their one-and-only true love. Picture five feisty, very-old-ladies in cotton smocks, some in wheelchairs, sitting in a circle, false-teeth rattling, bifocals slipping off noses, improvising this dialogue, and laughing a lot:

Sound effects: Slightly out-of-tune melodeon playing The Old Rugged Cross, *Women sobbing loudly.*

Anna: *Oh, my God! My beloved has passed away. I don't want to live anymore. Please wake up! This must be a bad dream. Please wake up! I don't want to live without you.*

Edith: *Oh, my darling, what am I going to do without you? I have nobody now. I'm so lonely!*

Isabel: *He was such a good man. I was going to marry him. How will I ever find another man?*

Anna: *What do you mean, you were going to marry him? I was going to marry him! He took a thousand dollars of my money. He was going to build us a beautiful house.*

Edith: *Who are you? How dare you say you were going to marry him! He took two-thousand dollars from me. We were planning a honeymoon trip around the world.*

Isabel: *You women are all crazy. This man was going to marry me!*

Emma: *I'm sorry, but all you ladies are mistaken. This dear man was going to marry me. He would never have wasted money in such frivolous ways. He had an old, sick mother, and he borrowed money from me to pay her doctor's bills.*

Rose: *You women are all crazy or stupid. I don't know which.*

Anna: *What do you mean by that?*

Edith: *How dare you say a thing like that!*

Rose: *I knew this guy better than any of you. I didn't have any money to give him, but he was taking me on a trip with your money.*

Isabel: *He was going to marry you?*

Emma: *No, he was going to marry me!*

Anna: *He wasn't going to marry you, he was going to marry me!*

Rose: *You women are a bunch of ninnies! He was living in sin with me. He wasn't going to marry anyone, but he was taking me on a trip around the world.*

Edith: *Oh, no! I can't believe it. He betrayed me.*

Isabel: *He promised to marry me. I trusted him!*

Emma: *He was philandering with other women! He took all my money. My life is ruined.*

Anna: *I dreamed of such a happy life with him. If he hadn't died, he might have deserted me anyway.*

Edith: *I was so sure of him. Now, I learn he was seeing other women.*

Isabel: *I still can't believe he was cheating on me.*

Emma: *He was cheating on all of us.*

Anna: *What a terrible man he was!*

Edith: *Well, thank God he's gone. I wouldn't want that devil, marrying everybody. Who wants a man like that?*

Isabel: *Not me. I don't want him!*

Emma: *You can have him.*

Anna: *Good riddance to bad rubbish!*

Edith: *If he was alive, I'd fix his wagon. I'd put pins in his bed!*

Isabel: *I'd cook his meals full of pepper and let him choke.*

Emma: *I'd make a voodoo doll and stick lots of pins in it. I'd make him suffer!*

Anna: *I'd put the bastard in jail!*

Edith: *I'd kill him. I'd boil him in oil!*

Rose: *You women are still being stupid. I'm just going to get myself another guy. I'm not going to sit around crying over him.*

Isabel: *She's right. I'm going to look for a good man.*

Emma: *A good man is hard to find, but I'll keep looking.*

Anna: *There are lots of good fish in the sea.*

Edith: *I don't need a man to be happy. I can live happily-ever-after, all by myself.*

Rose: *Listen ladies, it sounds like this fellow took a lot of your money.*

Anna: *That's right! He took a thousand dollars from me.*

Edith: *He took two thousand from me.*

Rose: *Well look at him lying over there in the coffin. He looks so smart in his nice suit, with his gold cufflinks, his diamond stickpin, and his fancy rings. There might be some money in his pockets, too.*

Isabel: *I bought him one of those rings.*

Emma: *I bought him the diamond stickpin.*

Anna: *I bought him those gold cufflinks.*

Rose: *Wouldn't it be a shame if he took all those beautiful things to the grave?*

Edith: *I say we should take them back!*

Isabel: *I'm with you!*

Emma: *Let's go!*

Anna: *Here we go!*

Sound effects: Women screaming. Stamping feet. A wooden coffin being tipped over and crashing to the floor

Exercise: Discovering your Parent's Passion

What did your parent do for fun when he was young and healthy?

Can those activities be modified so he can still do them, and how?

What new activities might your parent become interested in?

•

If my father had lived longer, I might have taken his taped stories, transcribed them, added appropriate photographs, and made them into a book. He would have been thrilled to see his words in print. I believe that he was lucky, growing old and dying in the familiar surroundings of his own apartment.

The last weeks before his death, his dementia grew worse and he was becoming incontinent. Had he lived much longer, I may have had to put him into a nursing home.

From my examples above, you can see that a nursing home can become a pleasant residence, and preferable to leaving your parent home alone, in what may have become a dangerous environment. At any age, moving house can be unpleasant, and moving an aging parent into new surroundings can be traumatic.

Even if your parent has seen the nursing-home and agrees to the move, packing-up can be a challenge. Before my father's death, I hung family photos, wall-to-wall, in his living room. He loved them, and I imagined moving them to a nursing-home, making his new room look like his old room.

Elly, a retired art teacher in her eighties, lived in a house with her adult granddaughter, Ruth. Elly kept herself busy with painting and crafts projects while Ruth commuted to work in the city. One evening, Ruth was surprised to come home and find an empty Meals on Wheels container.

Grandma Elly explained that she had seen a TV commercial where a charming young Meals On Wheels delivery man came to an old lady's house, sang to her, and delivered her meal. Expecting a similar theatrical experience, Elly had signed herself up for Meals On Wheels. Expecting a handsome young man to sweep up the drive and serenade her, she was unpleasantly surprised to see a bent-over, elderly man shuffling up her icy walkway. He knocked on her door, gave her the meal, smiled, but didn't sing.

Day after day, her meals were delivered by frail-looking, elderly people. Her disappointment was compiled by her worry that the deliverers would slip on the ice and hurt themselves. After a while, Elly didn't even want to see the deliverers. She left a rusty bucket outside, attached with a string, and a note saying the meal should be left inside. Just to be sure the deliverer wouldn't see her, she stayed inside, pulled the string, and dragged her lunch indoors.

As Elly's health deteriorated, it was no longer safe for her to stay home alone. Several relatives in another state invited Elly to live with them, but she refused to leave her home. A nursing-home was under construction nearby, so I suggested that Ruth take her grandmother on a drive and check it out. Fortunately, Elly liked what she saw and agreed to move into the home.

All seemed well, until Ruth started helping her grandmother pack. Elly wanted to take everything she owned, including piles of dried-up marking pens, and boxes of rubbish, left over from her many crafts projects.

The arguments raged until Ruth was at her wit's end. Suddenly, Elly had become a different person. Her Three

Truths were:

1. Your parent's basic personality type.
Parent Type 4: Unreasonably demanding.
2. Your relationship to your parent.
Strained.
3. What your parent needs to feel validated and whole.
She needs to keep all her belongings, even the trash.

I knew that Elly's memory was not sharp enough to remember which items were taken to the nursing-home, and which left behind, so I suggested that Ruth prepare two sets of boxes. One set was for useful, necessary items, and the other for useless items to be thrown away.

The ruse worked.

Elly thought she had won and was taking everything. Once they got to the nursing home and unpacked the boxes, she never missed the items that had been thrown away.

Ruth did not want to tell her grandmother a lie. She had no choice. The lie injured no one and made the move possible.

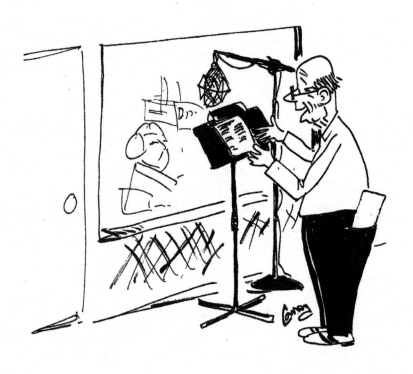

CHAPTER TEN
New Hobbies Reviving Old Passions

Passion is a curious thing. Three senior center members, at two different centers, discovered that their former jobs were actually their passions. These three men, Bill, Juan, and Sam were all retired and bored. They wanted something more in their lives, but didn't know what.

Bill contracted polio at the age of two and wore leg-braces his entire life. One of many children from a very poor family, he was never sent to regular public school, but instead, to an institution for physical and mental defectives. He was taught little academically, but did learn to grind eyeglasses, make costume jewelry, and earn a living.

When I met Bill, he was in his late sixties, shy, bored, and hanging around the senior center. He had little musical ability, but enjoyed singing in my chorus, and playing in the musical improvisation sessions I held once a week. Using portions of my Master's Degree Music Therapy thesis, the center received a generous music therapy grant.

I bought a wonderful array of exotic percussion instruments. Every week, a dozen center members gathered around my piano, improvised music and lyrics, sang, danced, pounded their drums, made lots of noise, and had a great time.

Trained musicians often have trouble improvising, because they worry about playing wrong notes. Unskilled musicians quickly enjoy the freedom of expression.

Improvising is playing music that has never been played before, so there are no wrong or right notes. Whatever sounds come out of the session are good sounds. No judgment!

After about a year of improvising, Bill and a few other center members came to me saying that they wanted to play, "real music." They wanted me to start a band. I was shocked, but intrigued. I carefully explained that playing "real music," meant they actually had to learn to play musical instruments, practice technique, take corrections, and learn the right notes. They were still adamant. I agreed and the band was formed.

I had a few gifted vocalists at the center, including three former WWII band singers. They were only interested in singing. The members who came to play in the band were not musically talented. This was a challenge. Using the band as accompaniment for the chorus, I arranged simple xylophone, recorder, one-hand keyboard, and percussion parts, and taught the members one by one.

I tried Bill on several instruments, and he finally settled on bass drum. He loved playing and his self-esteem grew. He became so proud of himself; he offered to teach a jewelry-making class. Before long, his class was a highlight of center activities. He had about a dozen elderly students. We were all buying and wearing his simple, attractive designs. His jewelry sales made money for the center, and he was suddenly a very important guy. If Bill had never tried playing a drum, he might never have gained the personal confidence to teach a jewelry-making class, rediscover his old passion, and create a product that benefited so many.

After eight years working at that senior center, I left to take over as director of a different senior center. Many of my elderly musicians followed me, and were quickly joined by new, elderly singers, dancers, and musicians. Some of the center members asked if I would teach them guitar and piano, and I was happy to oblige. Guitar players have to twist their left wrists in a very awkward position.

The fingers of their left hand need to push down very hard on thin nylon strings that cut into the flesh. It hurts. (I have a few elderly students who played guitar in their youth and preferred steel strings. All my beginners play nylon strings.)

Children can pick up guitar easily, but senior citizens with stiff joints usually have trouble. I had a dozen in my beginning guitar class, but half could not twist their wrists and bend their fingers tight enough to play. I encouraged them to switch to my recorder or piano classes. Both of those instruments are played with the hands and wrists in much more natural positions.

One gentleman who stayed in guitar class was Juan. Eighty-one, intelligent, well-educated, and very shy. He told me he loved many kinds of music, but he had never played a musical instrument. He had trouble making his stiff joints adapt to guitar technique, but he persevered. After months of disciplined practice, he learned to play a few first-position chords beautifully. Eventually, I had an instrumental ensemble of violin, recorders, keyboards, banjo, harmonics, concertina, and guitars. Juan played with the ensemble, got great joy from the music-making and socializing with the other players.

After he had played with my band for a couple of years, he told me that he was a Berlitz-trained Spanish teacher, and volunteered to teach a class at the senior center. Both his beginning and advanced level classes became so popular, he attracted new students to the center. If Juan had never studied guitar, he might never have gained the personal confidence to teach a Spanish class.

Another elderly gentleman, Sam, discovered that his old job was his passion. His first career was as an electrical engineer and his second as a psychotherapist.

When I first met him, he was in his late seventies and still seeing a few patients. Sam had never performed music or drama, but joined my senior center chorus, radio-drama group, and was instantly hooked. He was a natural-born ham.

Wanting more time in the spotlight, he offered to teach a lamp repair class. Every week, senior center members brought in their broken lamps, or other small appliances. If they wanted to learn, Sam taught them the basics of electrical repair. If they were not interested in learning, he fixed their appliances for the cost of the parts. One little-old-lady student learned so well, she got herself a repair job at a local lamp store.

Learning a new skill can rekindle passion in an old one. If your parent does not have a passion, try getting him interested in a hobby he has never done before, never even thought of doing, which has no judgment attached to it. Like the gentlemen listed above, your parent's new hobby could become a passion and lead him back to an old passion he has set aside.

If he chooses to share his passion, it can ignite passionate joy in others.

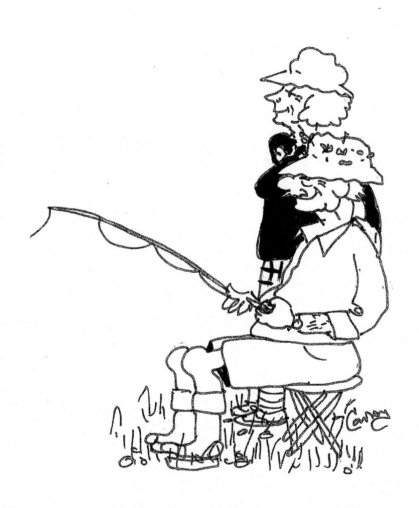

CHAPTER ELEVEN
A New Hobby becoming a Passion

A new passion can become a necessity we never knew we needed.

A few years ago a short, round lady shyly approached me. "I've always wanted to learn to play the piano, but I'm seventy-eight-years-old. Am I too old to learn?" Her big blue eyes looked up through a halo of thick, cropped white hair.

I smiled. "Of course you're not too old. You may never play well enough for Carnegie Hall, but you can certainly learn to play and have a lot of fun doing it."

"That makes me so happy!" Jane sighed with relief.

Two years later, Jane was eighty. She could play *Silent Night* and *Let me Call you Sweetheart* on the piano, with two hands. She recognized the meter and keys of the hymns she sang in church. She had also learned to play the recorder and performed simple parts in the musical arrangements I made for the senior center instrumental ensemble.

As a Certified Music Therapist, I had been teaching music to older adults for many years. Some came to me saying, "I took lessons as a child, but gave up and want to start again." If the student had a frame of reference, my job was easy. Jane had none. When she confided her fear that she might not be able to keep up with the class, my stomach tensed. This was going to be tough.

I explained that several students learned at once, each using his/her own keyboard, and listening through earphones. The keyboards were placed around a large room, and each student worked individually, at his/her own pace.

I went from student to student, spending a few minutes with each, then leaving them to practice as I went to the next.

Jane was eager to start. It was slow going. She had a slight hearing problem and a memory deficit typical to people her age. I would re-explain something for a fifth time, and she would say, "Oh, that's so interesting. I never knew that before." Slowly... so ... slowly ... she began to remember and learn.

Jane's children were so proud of her; they bought her a piano-keyboard. She was thrilled, then quickly overwhelmed by all the rows of tiny buttons, lights, numbers, and switches, the manufacturer installed so teenagers can play multiple styles of rock and rap. She could not figure out which buttons to push to make it play the simple sounds she needed.

This is a constant problem. Every piano keyboard model is different from every other. I am a professional musician, and I have to read each instruction book to figure out all the functions. Some amateurs find it impossible.

Every time one of my elderly students buys a keyboard, I end up at his/her apartment, reading the instruction book and figuring out how it works. When I visited Jane, she took careful notes of her keyboard's functions, so she could program it after I left.

One day, after a lesson, Jane became tearful. "You know, learning music has changed my life."

In a half-whisper, she told me she was a widow and had recently buried one of her children. Feeling sad and lonely, she had tried distracting herself by attending other senior programs. The activities were pleasant, but every night, she went home and sat in front of her TV—alone.

She said, "Now that I found your classes, I go home at night and practice the piano. A whole hour will go by and I won't even know it. I can't wait to play *All of Me* for my grandson." Jane never knew she needed music in her life. Once music became her passion, she couldn't live without it.

Ted was ninety and quite deaf when he came to my piano class. He was highly intelligent, and occasionally came late for practice because he was busy, trading online. He played piano in his youth, but when he lost his hearing, he thought his musical life was over.

I taught him to use a drum machine, so he was able to feel the rhythms and play keyboard with the ensemble. Rehearsing and performing with the group became his reason for living.

Occasionally, he accompanied singers, and I always warned the soloists they could not make any mistakes. Ted felt the drumbeat, but couldn't hear the singers. If they missed a beat, Ted just played on.

Ted always knew that his passion was music. He grieved its loss when he lost his hearing. I gave music back to him. Music gave him back his life.

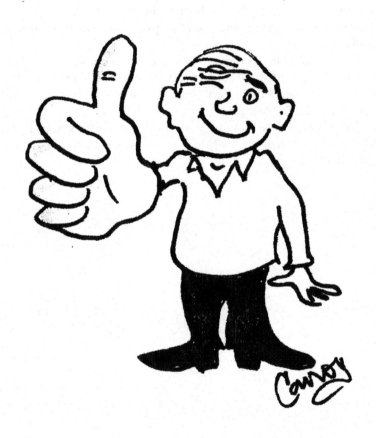

CHAPTER TWELVE
Shedding Healthy Tears

"When tears are not allowed to fall, inner organs weep."
Embroidered on a sampler dated 1886.

There is a song from Sweet Charity called, *I Love to Cry at Weddings.*

We love to cry happy tears for other people. We also love "three-Kleenex movies," that are "real tearjerkers."

I think we love to cry at made-up stories, because we can release the tension of tears without touching our own, personal pain. Shedding surrogate tears relaxes us, while causing us minimal distress.

During my training as a music therapist, I learned to deal with my patients' raw emotions. I encouraged them to express their fears and sorrows by crying, shouting, singing loudly, pounding on a piano, drums, or cymbals. It was sometimes scary, but always rewarding.

I will never forget a wheelchair-bound woman who came to the senior center for chair-exercise classes. Liz had suffered terrible strokes. Her face was so distorted she could barely speak. Whenever I greeted her, she looked up from her chair, smiled a terribly twisted smile back to me, but we had no other contact.

One day I walked past the exercise class and stopped dead. Liz was in her wheelchair, with her leg raised straight up. Her knee was against her nose. This was an agile pose for a trained athlete, let alone a woman who couldn't walk.

Very curious, I approached her at lunch and complimented her agility. With strained, hardly intelligible words, she told me that she had been a professional figure skater and a fashion model. I was fascinated, and she was flattered by my attention.

A few days later, I took her into a small room to play some music and see what might happen. We talked, as much as she was able. I played the piano, but neither of us remembered the tune to the *Skater's Waltz*. I improvised some other waltzes. She smiled and moved to the music, in her chair.

Suddenly, the tune came to me and I played the *Skater's Waltz*. Liz burst into loud, tragic, uncontrollable sobbing. Feeling terrible, I gave her some Kleenex and apologized for making her cry.

Eventually, she stopped crying and said that she was all right. Thinking I had done something horribly cruel, I wheeled her into lunch, and beat myself up for the rest of the day.

The next morning I saw Liz getting wheeled into the center and guiltily avoided her. During lunch, I noticed a group of seniors and staffers gathered around a lunch table. Moving in closer, I saw that Liz had brought in scrapbooks from her careers as a figure skater and fashion model. She proudly showed them off, and enjoyed the approval of the others.

When Liz saw me, she waved proudly and pushed the books over for me to see. What I thought had been cruel, had actually been kind. Without that emotional breakthrough, the day before, Liz never would have told anyone about her accomplishments, and gained self-esteem from our affirmations.

Liz never wanted the pain of crying, but she needed the emotional release. Once she was able to cry over her lost beauty and mobility, she was able to seek validation for the beautiful, graceful athlete she had once been.

Earlier, I wrote about Peter, the henpecked husband, care-taking his wife Emma. Peter's life was filled with genuine sadness and anger that he had never expressed. He was eighty-two, and still believed that big boys didn't cry.

Withholding his tears gave him stomach pain, appetite loss, headaches, and insomnia. I feared this could lead to a stroke or worse. His physical and vocal affects were so stiff, polite, and correct, that they were void of any real emotion.

During an individual music therapy session, he talked about his frustrations, but insisted that he could handle everything. His life was just fine.

I knew that he was not fine, and without a breakthrough, he would have a breakdown. Since he was a devout Catholic, I played church organ music on my keyboard while he spoke about the sadness in his life.

He tried keeping up his manly facade, but the music was more powerful than he was.

Finally, he burst into tears. I was relieved, and he was embarrassed. I handed him a box of Kleenex, kept playing, and let him cry. A few minutes later, he sat back, exhausted.

His eyes were red, but his body was more relaxed than I had ever seen it. After that, he cried in every therapy session he attended, group and individual.

The group members appreciated his emotional release, and praised his courage and tenacity, taking care of Emma.

I was pleased to see him looking relaxed, participating in more center activities, and knowing that I might have helped him to live longer.

Peter never wanted the pain of crying, but he needed to express his sadness. The emotional release allowed others to validate him, and tell him he had done well, taking care of Emma. He was finally able to really hear their compliments and appreciate how good a man he really was.

One of my nursing-home patients was a beautiful, gracious woman who had suffered a series of debilitating strokes.

Jenny had trouble speaking, was in constant pain, and heavily medicated. She had few visitors, and was physically incapable of attending group activities.

She often lay in bed, sobbing quietly.

The entire staff was kind and consoling, but nothing

seemed to comfort her.

One day I tried something very simple. I took my small harp to her bedside and quietly sang the folk song, *Kumbaya*.

She always loved my songs and the soothing tones from my harp. After singing a couple of conventional verses:

"Kumbaya, my Lord, Kumbaya ... and
Someone's praying Lord, Kumbaya ..."

I improvised,
"Someone's hurting Lord, Kumbaya,
Someone's hurting Lord, Kumbaya ..."

Her eyes popped wide open.

She nodded frantically and grunted, "Yes! Yes!"

Suddenly, she believed that I understood her pain. I kept singing as she smiled, and cried, and repeated, "Yes! Yes!"

Finally, she felt validated. Other staffers had sincerely told her they knew she was in pain, but it was my sung words,

"Someone's hurting Lord, Kumbaya ..." that finally resonated in her mind, released her frustration, and allowed her to believe I really, really understood her pain.

When I finished singing, she told me how grateful she was, awkwardly squeezed my hand, and lay back smiling.

When I was growing up, my mother and I had a typically strained mother/daughter relationship.

We had never talked honestly about anything important. When she was dying of cancer, we were both afraid to talk about death, so we made phony small-talk instead.

Whenever I left her bedside and got back to my solitary apartment, I cried alone. She probably cried alone, too. We should have cried together.

After she died, my father, brother, and I did not talk about death. We did not know how to relate and share our pain. We all cried alone.

Years later, I studied psychodrama and worked through some painful issues with my mother.

Then I cried in public, a lot. Some of my classmates were working through issues with their living parents. I urged them to work face to face while they still had the chance.

However troublesome your parent may be, you may still be able to improve that relationship. Grab the chance now.

It will not be here forever.

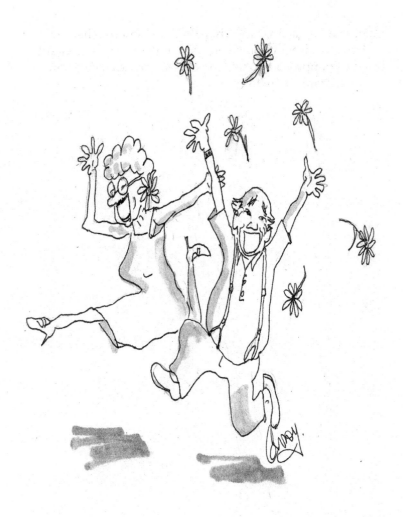

CHAPTER THIRTEEN
Enjoying Today

"I want to grow old, very old. It sure beats the alternative."

None of us are going to get out of this life alive. We don't know when or how we are going to die, so we may as well enjoy every day to the fullest. Your aging parent will probably go before you will, so enjoy him, while you have him. If you have never had fun together, start now!

First, figure out these Three Truths:

1. Your parent's basic personality type.
2. Your relationship to your parent.
3. What your parent needs to feel validated and whole.

After you have done that, use your imagination to find his passions. If he doesn't have a passion, find him a hobby. His new hobby may become a passion, or reawaken interest in an old passion. You may think his passion is silly, like my father talking about himself, day after day. It didn't matter what I thought. That activity made him happy. That was his passion. It didn't have to be mine.

Use your imagination and be tolerant. If your parent tells you he's in Lithuania … fine! He's in Lithuania.

Stay playful, relax a lot, and chances are the two of you will actually have fun together.

REFERENCES

Adult Day Care Centers

Respite Programs

Senior Citizen Centers

Settlement Houses

Lists of these state and local agencies are available online, at libraries, medical facilities, and through the following:
American Association of Retired Persons
National Council on Aging
National Institute on Aging
National Stroke Foundation
US Administration on Aging
Department for the Aging
National Institute of Health
Aging Research Center
Stage Offices on Aging
Elder Care
Alzheimer's Association
Family Caregiver Alliance
Alliance For Aging Research
US Senate Special Committee on Aging

BIBLIOGRAPHY

Bright, R. *Music in Geriatric Care.* Wahrooga, NSW 2076 Australia: Music Therapy Enterprises. 1991.

Brotons, M. & Pickett-Cooper, P. "Preferences of Alzheimer's disease patients for music activities: Singing, instruments, dance/movement, games and composition/ improvisation." *Journal of Music Therapy,* 1994. 21 (3), 220-233.

Clair, A.A. *Therapeutic Uses of Music with Older Adults.* Baltimore: Health Professional Press Inc. 1996.

Clair, A. A. & Ebberts, A. G. "The effects of music therapy on interactions between family caregivers and their care receivers with late stage dementia." *Journal of Music Therapy,* 1997. 33, (3), 148-164.

Cohen, G.D. *The Creative Age. Awakening human potential in the second half of life.* NY: Avon Press. 2000. Chapter 3, pp. 67-114.

Davis, W.B. "Music Therapy and Elderly Populations" in W.B. Davis, K.E. Gfeller & M.H. Thaut (Eds.) *An Introduction to Music Therapy, Theory, and Practice.* Boston: Mc-Graw-Hill College. 1999.

Dass, Ram. *Still Here: Embracing Aging, Changing, and Dying.* New York: Riverhead Books. 2000.

Digeronimo, Theresa Foy. *How to Talk to Your Senior Parents About Really Important Things: Specific Questions and Answers and Useful Things to Say.* San Francisco: Jossey-Bass. 2001.

Feil, N. *Validation / How to Help Disoriented Old-Old.* St. Louis, MO: MMB Music, Inc. 1989.

Gibson, H.B. *Loneliness in Later Life.* New York: St. Martin's Press. 2000.

Halstead, M. T. and Roscoe, S. T. "Restoring the Spirit at the End of Life: Music as an Intervention for Oncology Nurses." *Clinical Journal of Oncology Nursing: ONS Website.* 2004.

Hanson, N., Gfeller, K., Woodworth, G., Swanson, E.A. & Garand, L. "A comparison of the effectiveness of differing types and difficulty of music activities in programming for older adults with Alzheimer's disease and related disorders." *Journal of Music Therapy.* 1996. 23, (2), 93-123.

Lair, J. *I ain't much baby, but I'm all I've got.* United States of America: Fawcett Crest. 1972.

Lawton, P. and LaPorte, A. "Beyond Traditional Art Education: Transformative Lifelong Learning in Community-Based Settings with Older Adults: National Art Education Association, Studies in Art Education." *A Journal of Issues and Research.* 2013. 54 (4), 310-320.

Lipe, A. "The use of music performance tasks in the assessment of cognitive functioning among older adults with dementia." *Journal of Music Therapy.* 1995. 32, (3), 137-151.

Moore, R., Staum, M.J. & Brotons, M. "Music preferences of the elderly: Repertoire, vocal ranges, tempos, and accompaniments for singing." *Journal of Music Therapy.* 1992. 24, (4), 236-252.

Odell-Miller, H. "Why provide music therapy in the community for adults with mental health problems?" *British Journal of Music Therapy.* 1995. 9 (1), 4-10.

Kausler, Donald, H. and Kausler, Barry C. *The Graying of America: An Encyclopedia of Aging, Health, Mind, and Behavior.* Champaign, IL: University of Illinois Press. 2001.

Merriam, Sharan B. *Learning in Adulthood: A Comprehensive Guide.* San Francisco: Jossey-Bass-Reasd. 2007. Chapter 6 "Transformational Learning, pp 130-158.

Miller, P. A. "Interdisciplinary Teamwork: The key for quality care for older adults" in Tepper, L. M. and Cassidy, T. M. (eds.) *Multidisciplinary Perspectives on Aging.* NY: Springer Publishers. 2004. Chapter 16, 259-276.

Pipher, Mary Bray. *Another Country: Navigating the Emotional Terrain of Our Elders.* New York: Riverhead Books. 2000.

Pollack, N. J. & Namazi, K. H. "The effect of music participation on the social behavior of Alzheimer's disease patients." *Journal of Music Therapy.* 1992. 24, (1), 54-67.

Redinbough, E.M. "The use of music therapy in developing a communication system in a withdrawn, depressed older adult resident: A case study." *Music Therapy Perspectives.* 1988. 5, 82-85.

Short, A.E. "Insight-oriented music therapy with elderly residents." *The Australian Journal of Music Therapy.* 1995. 6, 4-18.

Rowe, John & Kahn, Robert. *Successful Aging.* New York: Pantheon Books. 1998.

Snowdon, David. *Aging with Grace: What the Nun Study Teaches Us About Leading Longer, Healthier, and More Meaningful Lives.* New York: Bantam Books. 2001.

CPSIA information can be obtained
at www.ICGtesting.com
Printed in the USA
FSOW04n1105190717
36312FS